A BEAUTIFUL SCAR

BEAUTY & MAKEUP TIPS ON HOW YOU CAN IMPROVE THE APPEARANCE OF YOUR SCAR

By

ESTHER CLAASEN

Copyright © 2015

Instagram #skin_series

INTRODUCTION

As a skin care professional with international qualifications, I have over twenty years of experience with the skin and have my own scar story to share.

Are you living with a scar and feel unhappy and self conscious? Do you feel that your everyday life is restricted due to you having a scar that looks unattractive?

Read on and learn some fantastic practical advice about how you can improve the condition and appearance of your scar.

TABLE OF CONTENTS

LEGAL NOTES

CHAPTER 1: MY STORY

My scar is smack bang on the right hand side of my chest sitting just above my heart. Reasonably large it measures 4.5 cm across and 6cm down, so quite obvious! As a young and rebellious 19 year old teenager I hung out with the wrong crowd and before we arrived at a concert, we all decided to get tattoos. A decision that I do not regret so much now however when I decided to turn my life around, move away from my old social circle my tattoo, a pretty purple flower, became a constant reminder of my not so proud moments. So I wanted to get rid of my tattoo fast.

In 1991 laser tattoo removal was not prevalent in New Zealand and I jumped in rather hastily and decided, with very little research or enough professional guidance, to have my tattoo removed surgically. While under general anesthetic the plastic surgeon cut out the tattoo and then removed skin from my upper inner thigh area and, used this piece of skin as a skin graft to replace the tattooed skin.

Under strict instructions from the plastic surgeon I kept the skin graft flat as possible using surgical tape and after a few weeks the tape was removed revealing a flat and very red looking wound. Now had I have done my research, and maybe listened to the plastic surgeon who warned me of bad scarring, I would have realized that keloid scarring is very high on the chest area, given the range of movement. At this point I realized that my head strong relentless determination and lack of foresight resulted in a change of course for me.

As time passed my scar started to take on an increasingly raised and red lumpy appearance. At it's worst the scarring was at least half a centimeter raised above my chest and, as you can imagine put me in a state of extreme distress. In haste I immediately rang the plastic surgeon's office and cried out that the implications of potentially bad scarring were not properly explained to me. As a result I refused to pay for the balance of the operation and they never asked for it either. This is probably where I wished that my parents had of interceded more and refused the operation and made me wait for better methods of scar removal. However were my parents and the doctors really to blame? Looking back I should have listened more to the advice of the people around me.

Never one to sit still I set about on researching the best methods of scar therapy that was available to me and this book is a record of how I improved the condition and appearance of my scar and how I came to terms with the fact that you can never permanently remove a scar and there is no miracle laser that will make them disappear. It is my hope that this book will encourage you and reiterate that it is better to do something practical about your situation than to sit around and feel sad about it. Although my scar was small in comparison to others who are affected with much larger scars the emotional pain can still be just as strong and a desire to improve the scar no less.

CHAPTER 2: TYPES OF SCARS

Scars are areas of fibrous tissue that replace normal skin after an injury and a scar results from the process of wound repair in the skin and other tissues of the body. Scarring is a natural part of the healing process and with the exception of very minor lesions every wound results in some degree of scarring.

HYPERTROPHIC SCAR

Hypertrophic scars occur when the body overproduces collagen, which then causes the scar to be raised above the surrounding skin. Hypertrophic scars take the form of a red raised lump on the skin. They usually occur within 4 to 8 weeks following wound infection or wound closure with excess tension and/or other traumatic skin injuries.

KELOID SCAR

Keloid scars are inert masses of collagen and are completely harmless and not cancerous; however they can be itchy or painful in some individuals. Keloid scars can occur on anyone but they are most common in people with a darker skin colour and generally occur on the shoulders and chest (high movement's areas). Keloid scarring can be caused by surgery, accident, acne or, sometimes, body piercings.

ATROPHIC SCAR

An atrophic scar takes the form of a sunken recess in the skin, which has a pitted appearance. These are caused when underlying structures supporting the skin, such as fat or muscle are lost. This type of scarring is often associated with acne, chickenpox or other diseases such as Staphylococcus, surgery, or accidents.

STRETCH MARK SCAR

Stretch marks, are caused when the skin is stretched rapidly like during pregnancy, significant weight gain, or adolescent growth spurts or when skin is put under tension during the healing process, usually near joints. This type of scar can improve in appearance after a few years. Sometimes stretch marks will start as red/purple in appearance and fade to white/silver over time.

IMMATURE/MATURE SCARS

The maturity of scars is not determined by the age of them. Some abnormal scars remain active and therefore immature for very long periods of time. A good way of identifying those are through symptoms. Pain, inelasticity or general discomforts are key symptomatic features of immature scars. There can also be dermatological signs such as redness, hyper/hypo-pigmentation and elevated skin from the scar. My scar can now be described as mature, flat and pale and I have found that over time the scar has blended into the surrounding skin.

CHAPTER 3: PRACTICAL STEPS TO IMPROVE THE APPEARANCE OF YOUR SCAR

HOME SKIN CARE

MASSAGE

Eight weeks after my skin graft surgery I developed a very raised, red and angry looking scar, a hypertrophic scar. Rather shocked and upset at such an ugly looking scar I immediately went into "practical survival" mode, and started a daily massage with a Vitamin E Cream.

Every evening without fail I gently massaged my scar for around 5 – 10 minutes and also used a very gentle baby tooth brush to help stimulate the cut nerve endings. Over time this massage helped to improve the colour of my scar, break down and flatten the collagen fibres and also promote some feeling in and around my scar, which in the early days was very numb.

This "ritualistic" routine continued for at least two years and I strongly believe that regular massage if advised by your doctor is performed then it can really improve the appearance of your scar forever. Still to this day twenty years on I will massage an oil or cream into my scar.

HOME CARE - LOTIONS AND POTIONS

Scars need a high degree of hydration to keep them supple and this continued suppleness aids in improving a scars appearance, especially when you have a good skin care routine.

I began my scar beauty routine by simply using all of my existing products for the face, and extending down onto my chest area. Day and night my scar would receive a cleansing, tone and moisturize with weekly gentle exfoliation, serums and hydration masks.

The following is your bathroom wish list to begin your scar skincare routine today;

Sunblock – Sun exposure on a scar can cause pigmentation or even worse sunburn. If exposing your scar always ensure that you apply and reapply a high protection non greasy sunscreen.

Rosehip Oil – Rosehip Oil is bursting with essential fatty acids, vitamins and antioxidants. Incredibly healing, apply rosehip oil to your scar as part of your evening skin care routine.

Coconut Oil – Coconut Oil is very rich in essential fatty acids and lubricates scars wonderfully. In the evening gently massage into your skin before you hop into the shower or apply on damp skin after your shower. I tend not to use oils in the morning as my sunblock does not sit so well.

Bio Oil – I have found great results with Bio Oil especially with my stretch-marks. Made from plant extracts and vitamins, this product has had extensive research and great results for all types of scarring.

Skin Brushing – I have recently started skin brushing with a natural bristle brush and it is great for stimulating the nerve endings in your skin, exfoliating dead skin, leaving you with a healthy glow.

Organic Body Moisturizer – You can use any brand really just as long as it is non-greasy and can sit well under your sunblock for your morning skin care routine.

Ok so what else worked for me?

STEROID INJECTIONS

In the early days my scar reacted very well to steroid injections and after only two sessions with an experienced and reputable plastic surgeon the redness, lumps and raised appearance virtually disappeared. Unfortunately my scar still remained and the pale colour from the line surrounding the skin graft very evident but hey at least I was on the right track!

Interestingly the same Plastic Surgeon also experimented with injecting a flesh tone pigment into the pale thin line to match up my scar with the skin colour of my chest. Unfortunately this procedure did not work as well as the pigment colour was not a good match (so hard to replicate nature I guess!) and the pigment faded over a short period of time.

Just so you know, loss of pigment is very common in scars and is due to the loss of melanocytes (skin colour producing cells) in the underlying tissues of your skin. Currently there is no product or procedure that can bring back your natural skin colour. Hopefully this will change one day soon.

OZONE THERAPY - ALTERNATIVE MEDICINE

In the early nineties I visited a local beauty clinic and started a series of Ozone Therapy Treatments to further improve the colour of my scar and stimulate the nerve endings. Although not used as widely now in beauty clinics Ozone Therapy, helps to increase the amount of oxygen through the body. After approximately five treatments I believe that the colour overall improved, especially the very pale and lifeless looking area in the middle of my skin graft and also helped to improve the numb feeling.

STRATADERM - MEDICATED CREAM

In 2011 a fantastic dermatologist highly recommended Strataderm to further improve the appearance of my scar. Used daily the Strataderm formed a silicone sheet over my scar which helped to reduce dehydration, and improved the hydration of the underlying tissue. Applied sparingly for around two months the edges of my scar appeared smoother and the colour more healthy. Please note that Strataderm can cause redness and it did with me after a while but the redness goes very quickly.

You can purchase Strataderm online or at your local chemist.

MICROSKIN

Microskin is a simulated second skin that is formulated individually to colour correct scars or skin conditions such as loss of pigmentation. I went for a great consultation to their Brisbane Clinic and the product is sprayed on like a second skin and once dry is waterproof and durable. Let's be honest, its expensive however does a great job if you have the budget and you scar is wide spread or you cannot find a camouflage product with a skin colour to suit. This can be bought online.

CHAPTER 4: NUTRITION AND SCARRING

I am a big believer in you are what you eat and a healthy diet that includes a variety of nutrient-rich foods is vital. Whether you have a newly formed scar or a more mature scar your skin is always in need of nourishment and extra help.

I believe that a well-balanced healthy diet low on processed food captures most of the vital nutrients Plenty of fruit and vegetables, especially leafy greens and I absolutely love avocados – very rich in good fats, vital for skin health. Lean meats and fish with a handful of nuts or seeds are essentially on my hit list as well as plenty of water. And of course there is nothing wrong with a bit of a sweet chocolate treat – just for that feel good factor.

Just so you know when you are wandering down the supermarket isles, scars specifically require the following dietary nutrients to heal well:

- **Protein** – This helps the body create new tissue, especially collagen. They also improve the immune system which can fight off infections – Look for lean meats, fish, tofu, nuts (especially pumpkin seeds), greek yogurt, lentils, peanut butter, cottage cheese and eggs.

- **Vitamin C** – for healthy collagen production. Look for chilli peppers, red and green capsicum, kale, broccoli, papaya, strawberries, cauliflower, brussel sprouts, pineapple, kiwi fruit and mango.

- **Vitamin B Complex** – speeds up wound healing and helps to prevent inflammation. Look for potatoes, leafy greens such as spinach, asparagus, lentils, dried beans, peas, peanuts, butternut pumpkin, pork, fish, sunflower seeds and avocado.

- **Vitamin A** – activates production of connective tissue, including collagen, and helps new blood vessels grow to nourish newly formed tissue. Vitamin A also enhances resistance to infection by stimulating the body's immune system. Look for sweet potato, carrots, kale, butternut pumpkin, dried apricots, rock–melon, red capsicum, fish and mango

- **Zinc** – reduces healing time after surgery by up to 43% and can also reduce inflammation and bacterial growth. Look for Oysters (not necessarily an everyday ingredient!), fortified cereals such as bran, wholegrain, multigrain cereals, red meat, pork, wheatgerm, pumpkin seeds, spinach, nuts, cocoa and chocolate, avocados, blueberries, pomegranates.

CHAPTER 5: LAZER THERAPY

I never received laser treatment for my scar probably because it was not an option in the early 1990s due to the high cost and the technology was not as advanced as it is today. To help you in your quest for scar improvement I researched what is currently on offer.

Please note that I strongly advise that you consult a plastic surgeon or a highly experienced dermatologist referred to you by a doctor. In the wrong hands lasers can cause more harm than good. And please be aware that there are potential side effects such as redness, infection, bruising, sun sensitivity, scarring and extended healing time.

Pulsed Dyed Lasers – Early Scars, Older Scars & Red Stretch Marks

Pulsed dyed lasers deliver an intense burst of light into the skin which is absorbed by specific blood vessels or melanin pigmented areas. This type of laser can improve the colour, texture and pliability of scar tissue.

Fractional Lasers – Post Traumatic Scars and Acne Scars

Fractional laser uses light energy to create thousands of microscopic channels in the skin which are surrounded by areas of healthy, untreated skin. The zones of untreated skin allow for faster healing and make it more suitable for patients of darker skin type (in contrast to older resurfacing technologies that treated one hundred percent of the skin's surface.) The treated areas stimulate production of new collagen, plumping up the skin and smoothing out wrinkles, lines, scars and other irregularities.

Ablative Laser – more invasive, good for acne scarring and pigmentation irregularities

During ablative laser resurfacing, an intense beam of light energy (laser) is directed at your skin. The laser beam destroys the outer layer of skin (epidermis). At the same time, the laser heats the underlying skin (dermis), which causes collagen fibers to shrink. As the wound heals, new skin forms that's smoother and tighter.

Non-ablative Laser

Nonablative Laser damages collagen beneath your skin and stimulates the growth of new collagen, tightening underlying skin and improving skin tone and appearance. No skin is removed.

Your doctor will apply a thick ointment to the treated skin and might cover the area with an airtight and watertight dressing. To relieve pain after the procedure, take an over-the-counter pain reliever and apply ice packs.

Laser Tattoo Removal

Given my story I thought it fitting to provide a little information about removing your tattoo safely and with minimal scarring. The lasers now used to remove tattoos deliver ultra-short bursts of energy to the skin and shatter the pigments which are then easily eliminated by your body. Now before you get excited there are many factors that need to be taken into consideration, such as age of tattoo, pigments used, and possible skin reactions to the lazer. There can also be some very faint markings left once the lazer sessions have been completed. One to three sessions are generally necessary. **And please I implore you do your own research and find a reputable operator, as in the wrong hands can lead to scarring.**

CHAPTER 6: EASY CAMOUFLAGE MAKE UP TIPS

THE ART OF CAMOUFLAGE

I have experimented with camouflage make up over the years with mixed results however the technology now used to create these types of products are fantastic!

I currently use Dermablend and it's formulations have really improved over the years. This product used in conjunction with the techniques that I learnt from a consultant at the Microskin Institute in Brisbane has resulted in my following top eight camouflage make up tips.

If you have a smaller scar or a wider spread scar, such as a burn, correctly applied camouflage makeup enables you to wear clothing that you have had hidden in your wardrobe for years. I live In Noosa where going to the beach is a way of life all year round, so being able to wear low cut swimsuits has been an incredible confidence booster to me.

1. The success of your camouflage will largely depend on the condition of your skin before starting. Exfoliate on a regular basis and moisturize, this way your skin will be supple and smooth, providing a perfect canvas to apply your camouflage make up.

2. Ensure you remove gently any body hair that is on the area. As the light will pick up the tiny hairs and be very noticeable once the make-up is applied. I gently use a razor to remove the super fine hair on my chest. This grows very slowly and I do not have to do this all of the time. My hair is super fine and blonde, however if your hair is thicker then laser hair removal or waxing may be more a suitable option.

3. If you are going out in the day I recommend using an spf lotion 30. Use one that is not too greasy and will absorb easily into your skin. Avoid the lotions that are called dry touch as these are not hydrating enough on the skin. Alternatively if you are going out at night use a light hydrating lotion that is not too greasy and easily absorbed.

4. Take your camouflage product and pop a little onto the back of your hand. Dermablend have a variety of colours. For my fair skin colour I use the Dermablend Beige colour and have the

tawny colour for extra colour in the height of summer with my natural tan. With your index finger gently warm the product and start applying to the area that you want to cover using an up and down motion, not circular as this does not give an even finish. Now the secret to good scar coverage is to extend the area of your makeup. For example I camouflage my whole chest area, this way you have a very even skin tone otherwise if you just cover your scar there will be a more noticeable finish.

5. Now with good lighting apply small amounts each time over an area surrounding your scar. As you go blend the outer areas into your skin gently. You will notice that the warmth of your fingertips and body warmth will help the blending process. Once complete have a good look and then let dry for around the recommended time. This is a very important step in the process as if you apply powder before your makeup is dry your finish will not be as professional looking.

6. Once dry get your powder applicator and press your setting powder into your skin, a firm pressing movement will ensure the powder adheres to your makeup. Any excess you can gently brush off with clean and dry hands.

7. You are now ready to go and enjoy life and when you are ready to remove product simply apply in gentle circular motions your facial cleanser to remove and hydrate with a body oil and or body moisturizer.

8. I find that at the beach, while the makeup does cover your scar if it is not completely smooth away from direct light the shadows will reveal some of the unevenness of your skin. This sounds very silly but I will head to the beach in the cooler months when the sun is higher in the sky as the light reflects off my makeup and my scar is virtually undetectable!! The evening can be great too for lighting, especially in restaurants if the lighting is dim you can wear low cut tops or silk shirts to your heart content!!

CHAPTER: Fashion and Scars

Once I realized that no treatment in the world was ever going to remove my scar, I vowed to enjoy and celebrate my love of fashion. Here are my top five tips when you really need to plan your wardrobe according to where your scar is on your body and also improve your confidence.

1. Find a good tailor. Do not hesitate taking your clothes to be tailored for concealing your scars. As mine is in quite an obvious place on my chest I quite often take up straps or adjust a neckline.

2. Dress practically and manage your time. Go for items that cover your scar if possible especially if you are racing out of the door! I generally use my camouflage makeup when going to the beach or out for special occasions. If you have a scar that you cannot hide allow enough time to cover with your makeup.

3. Choose fabrics wisely. If you have a scar on your body chances are your skin may be a little sensitive. Go for the more natural fabrics

such as cotton, silk, viscose, linen, cashmere. Your skin will breathe.

4. Look good and feel good. I vowed that because of my scar I would invest time into looking great in fashion! I discovered that classic pieces really last. Nothing beats a classic white tee-shirt or shirt teamed up with a great pair of jeans or tailored shorts and a blazer. Finish off with a good quality pair of ballet flats and off you go!

5. Be Wary of Trends! If a certain seasonal trend does not suit you, such as leopard print then stay clear and stick to your own personal style. If you do not know your own style and you can afford one get a professional stylist to help you.

CHAPTER 7: HOW DOES YOUR SCAR MAKE YOU FEEL?

At the time of writing this book I asked a plastic surgeon if she could improve my scar. The surgeon took one look and said given the area, my scar is fantastic looking and the original surgeon did a wonderful job with the skin graft – much to my disbelief! Sometimes you just need a word of encouragement to make you realize how far you have come. Had I not taken matters into my own hands and used practical measures to help heal my scar, the surgeon's comments may not have been so positive.

I fully understand what it is like to suffer emotionally as a result of a scar. In the early days I would pray so hard that when I woke up my scar would magically disappear and given that my scar was on a very feminine area, this affected me very deeply and had an impact on my daily life.

I was not able to wear swimsuits and frolic on the beach with my friends or wear low cut dresses to cocktail parties. Neither could I embark on a relationship in the normal carefree way as the thought of my scar suddenly being discovered nor was a look of disgust on the face of others at times just too hard to bear.

Of course popular culture does not make it easy on those of us who have scars that make us feel self-conscious. We are bombarded with images of flawless models (most often photo shopped!) with perfect bodies which only serve as a reminder of our imperfections. So I say to you try and avoid buying or looking at literature which only makes you feel bad about yourself and concentrate on filling your mind with plenty of positive stuff. What interests you? Cooking, Sport, Books, Music, Current Affairs? You may find that over time you will become emotionally stronger and more confident so that these types of images may no longer hurt your feelings. And most importantly if you are feeling unhappy about your scar, do something practical today. Start by talking with a trusted family member, medical professional or friend.

The End

ABOUT THE AUTHOR

ESTHER CLAASEN is an internationally qualified skin care professional with over twenty years experience.

With a degree in English Literature and Business I have combined my interest in the skin and writing, in between being a busy partner and mummy to bring you my first book in The Skin Series.

OTHER BOOKS BY ESTHER CLAASEN

I am currently writing my second book in The
Skin Series – watch this space!

www.ingramcontent.com/pod-product-compliance
Lightning Source LLC
Chambersburg PA
CBHW062030280526
45787CB00005B/2274

ISBN 9781517487980

9000

Essential Oils For Weight Loss, Stress Relief, Aromatherapy, Beauty Care, Easy Recipes For Health and Beauty

Essential Oils

GUIDE

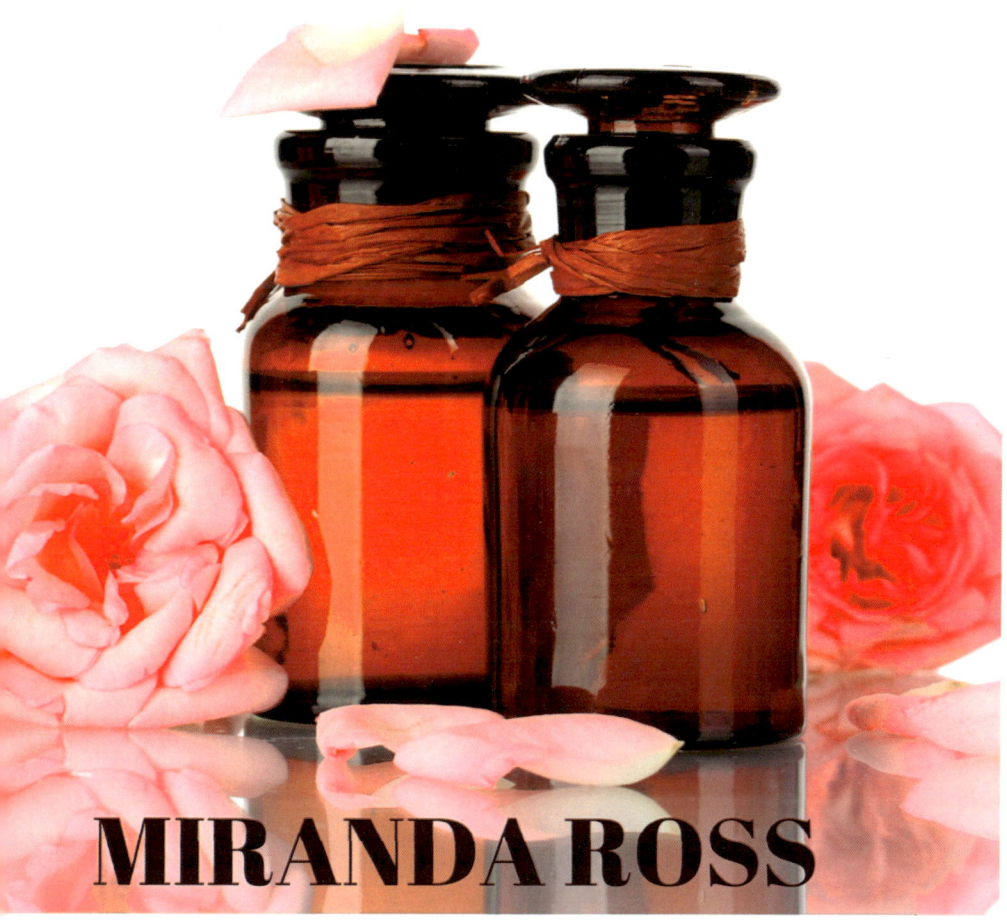

MIRANDA ROSS